Department of Economic and Social Affairs
Population Division

ST/ESA/SER.A/299

World Population Monitoring
Focusing on Health, Morbidity, Mortality
and Development

A Concise Report

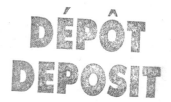

DÉPÔT
DEPOSIT

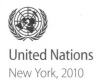

United Nations
New York, 2010

DESA

The Department of Economic and Social Affairs of the United Nations Secretariat is a vital interface between global policies in the economic, social and environmental spheres and national action. The Department works in three main interlinked areas: (i) it compiles, generates and analyses a wide range of economic, social and environmental data and information on which Member States of the United Nations draw to review common problems and to take stock of policy options; (ii) it facilitates the negotiations of Member States in many intergovernmental bodies on joint courses of action to address ongoing or emerging global challenges; and (iii) it advises interested Governments on the ways and means of translating policy frameworks developed in United Nations conferences and summits into programmes at the country level and, through technical assistance, helps build national capacities.

Note

The designations employed and the presentation of the material in this publication do not imply the expression of any opinion whatsoever on the part of the Secretariat of the United Nations concerning the legal status of any country, territory, city or area or of its authorities, or concerning the delimitation of its frontiers or boundaries.

The term "country" as used in the text of this publication also refers, as appropriate, to territories or areas.

The designations "more developed", "less developed" and "least developed" for countries, areas or regions are intended for statistical convenience and do not necessarily express a judgement about the stage reached by a particular country or area in the development process.

ST/ESA/SER.A/299

UNITED NATIONS PUBLICATION

Sales No. E.10.XIII.10

ISBN 978-92-1-151476-6

Preface

In resolution 1955/55 of 28 July 1995, the Economic and Social Council endorsed the terms of reference and the topic-oriented and prioritized multi-year work programme proposed by the Commission on Population and Development at its twenty-eighth session.[1] According to the multi-year work programme, which has served as the framework for assessment of progress made in implementing the Programme of Action of the International Conference on Population and Development,[2] a new series of reports on a special set of themes would be prepared annually. The Commission, in its decision 2008/101, established that the special theme for its forty-third session would be "health, morbidity, mortality and development". This report is a revised version of the report presented to the Commission at its forty-third session.

This report documents the major reductions in mortality achieved since 1950 in all countries and the shifting burden of disease from communicable to non-communicable diseases. It also documents how that shift has entailed a change in the age profile of mortality, from one in which a major proportion of deaths occur before age five to another where most deaths occur at older ages (above age 60). Because the majority of non-communicable diseases are chronic, persons suffering from them require long-term treatment. The successful management and treatment of the growing number of cases of chronic disease requires a comprehensive primary health-care approach, which integrates individual and population-based care by blending the clinical skills of physicians with epidemiology, preventive medicine and health promotion. Prevention is essential to reduce the burden of non-communicable diseases and it entails, in particular, the promotion of healthy diets and exercise as well as the reduction of tobacco use and the prevention of alcohol abuse. A well-functioning primary health-care system is also necessary to achieve the health-related Millennium Development Goals. To ensure universal access to the health system, the report suggests that health-care coverage be expanded by pooling resources and by implementing prepayment schemes.

On the basis of its deliberations at its forty-third session, the Commission on Population and Development adopted Resolution 2010/1 on

---

[1] See *Official Records of the Economic and Social Council, 1995, Supplement No. 7* (E/1995/27), annex 1, sects. I and III.

[2] *Report of the International Conference on Population and Development, Cairo, 5-13 September 1994* (United Nations publication, Sales No. E.95.XIII.18), chap. 1, resolution 1, annex.

"Health, morbidity, mortality and development". The full text of the resolution is presented in an annex to this report.

This report was prepared by the Population Division of the Department for Economic and Social Affairs of the United Nations Secretariat. For more information, please contact Hania Zlotnik, Director, Population Division, United Nations, New York, NY 10017, U.S.A.

Contents

		Page
Introduction		1
I.	Mortality trends	3
II.	Causes of death	9
III.	The burden of disease	13
IV.	Health and development	17
V.	The role of primary health care	21
VI.	The need for health workers	25
VII.	Prevention and treatment of communicable diseases and maternal conditions	27
VIII.	Prevention of non-communicable diseases	31
IX.	Preventing injuries	37
X.	Conclusions and recommendations	39
Annex		43

Table

I.	Distribution of disability adjusted life years according to cause for the world and income groups, 2004	14

Figures

I.	Evolution of life expectancy at birth by income group and major area, 1950-1955 to 2005-2010	4
II.	Life expectancy at birth by sex for income and geographical groups, 1990-1995 and 2005-2010	5
III.	Under-five mortality by major area, 1950-1955 to 2005-2010	6
IV.	Probability of surviving to age 60 according to the mortality rates of 2005-2010 by sex and major area	7
V.	Distribution of deaths by age group and major area, 2005-2010	8
VI.	Distribution of deaths by cause and major area, 2004	9
VII.	Number of deaths by cause, sex and age group, 2004	10
VIII.	Percentage of deaths by cause for major income group, 2004	11
IX.	Distribution of disability adjusted life years by age group for the income groups, 2004	15
X.	The relationship of life expectancy at birth and GDP per capita, 1980-1985 and 2000-2005	17

Introduction

The unprecedented decrease in mortality that began to accelerate in the more developed parts of the world in the nineteenth century and expanded to all the world in the twentieth century is one of the major achievements of humanity. By one estimate, life expectancy at birth increased from 30 to 67 years between 1800 and 2005, leading to a rapid growth of the population: from 1 billion in 1810 to nearly 7 billion in 2010.

Over the past two centuries, decreasing mortality has generally been accompanied by rising incomes but there is agreement that advances in technology and in the understanding of the causes of disease are responsible for the major share of that decline. Thus, higher calorie intake made possible by rising agricultural productivity, better hygiene facilitated by improvements in sanitation and access to safe drinking water, the development of insecticides, and the many breakthroughs in medical technology leading to cost-effective public health interventions and effective treatments have all contributed to reduce the incidence of disease at younger ages and prevent death when disease strikes.

A major change in the causes of death underlies the decline in mortality. Low life expectancies are typical of populations where the majority of deaths are due to communicable diseases and mortality in childhood is high. Marked increases in longevity have resulted from controlling the spread of communicable diseases and using effective medicinal drugs to treat them. An epidemiological transition has thus occurred whereby the causes of death have passed from being preponderantly communicable diseases to being dominated by non-communicable diseases. Concomitantly, the distribution of deaths by age has shifted to older ages and life expectancy has reached unprecedentedly high levels.

In the 1970s, when it became clear that the major infectious and parasitic diseases that had affected humanity for centuries were being successfully controlled or treated, thus reducing mortality even in the absence of sustained economic growth, the expectation was that mortality from communicable diseases would continue to decline everywhere. The advent of the human immunodeficiency virus (HIV) dashed those hopes and introduced an era where increases in mortality due to communicable disease became a reality in many low-income countries. In addition, infectious agents have been found to be the root cause of diseases that are considered non-communicable, such as cancers of the cervix, liver or stomach, and the emergence of new infectious agents, such as severe acute respiratory syndrome (SARS), or the mutations of the influenza virus pose the threat of a world pandemic. Consequently, there are growing concerns that the decline in mortality may not continue in the future.

This report documents past trends in mortality, the changing causes of death and the burden of disease. It reviews our current understanding of the interrelations between health and development, and discusses the main health challenges facing countries at different stages of development. Improving health and reducing mortality is a major objective of development, as the Millennium Development Goals make plain. But, as this report will show, the health-related Millennium Development Goals focus on the causes of a small share of deaths worldwide and are relevant mainly for low-income countries. Major efforts are already under way to achieve the Goals and in 2009 the Commission on Population and Development focused its deliberations on their attainment.[3] For that reason, this report focuses mainly on health issues beyond the Millennium Development Goals and on measures to ensure that health improvements are achieved on all fronts.

---

[3] See the report of the Secretary-General on world population monitoring, focusing on the contribution of the Programme of Action of the International Conference on Population and Development to the internationally agreed development goals, including the Millennium Development Goals (E/CN.9/2009/3).

Chapter I
Mortality trends[4]

Globally, life expectancy increased rapidly after 1950, rising from 47 years in 1950-1955 to 68 years in 2005-2010. The largest gains were made by developing countries, whose average life expectancy rose from 41 to 66 years, but life expectancy increased in every region. As a result, gaps in life expectancy between major areas and among income groups narrowed. Nevertheless, major differences persist. Today's high-income countries[5] have higher life expectancies than the middle-income countries and life expectancy is lowest in low-income countries (figure I). Geographically, northern America and Europe have experienced the highest life expectancies and recorded the lowest increases since 1950, partly because they started from a high base. In addition, rising mortality in Eastern Europe, particularly in the Russian Federation, during the early 1980s and after 1990 dampened the rise in European life expectancy.

In the developing world, Asia recorded the highest gains in life expectancy since 1950, with China and India achieving major increases: from 41 and 38 years, respectively, in 1950-1955 to 72 and 68 years in 2005-2010. Life expectancy also rose considerably in Latin America and the Caribbean—from 51 to 73 years—especially after starting from a moderate level. Africa, however, had made only moderate progress by 1980 and, because of the HIV/AIDS epidemic, has not yet managed to lift its average life expectancy above 55 years. Because the low-income countries include India, recent improvements in life expectancy in that group have surpassed those in Africa and their average life expectancy has reached 60 years.

In all regions and income groups female life expectancy exceeds male life expectancy (figure II). Globally, females have a life expectancy of 70 years in 2005-2010, compared to 65 for males. The female advantage in life expectancy is highest in Europe and in Latin America and the Caribbean. In Europe, the large female advantage owes much to the markedly higher survivorship of females than males in Eastern Europe, particularly in the Russian Federation, where, at current mortality rates, females expect to live 13 years longer than males (73 v. 60 years). In Latin America and the Caribbean the female advantage amounts to 7 years of life expectancy. The female

[4] All estimates cited in this section are from *World Population Prospects: The 2008 Revision* (United Nations publication, Sales No. 09.XII.6).

[5] The list of countries by income group can be found in *The Global Burden of Disease: 2004 Update* (World Health Organization, 2008).

Figure I
**Evolution of life expectancy at birth by income group and major area,
1950-1955 to 2005-2010**

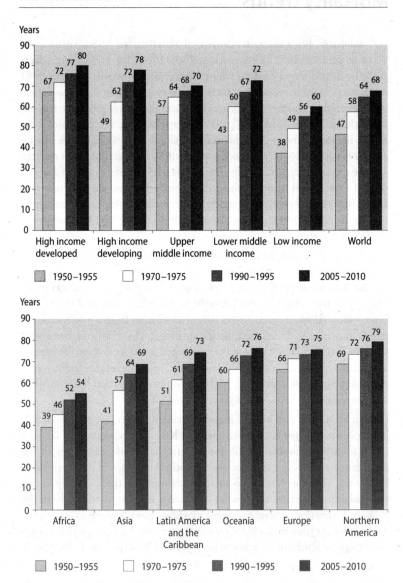

advantage is lowest in Africa, amounting to scarcely 2 years, partly as a result
of the high prevalence of HIV/AIDS among African women and high levels
of maternal mortality in the region. In all regions, except Asia, the female

Figure II
Life expectancy at birth by sex for income and geographical groups, 1990-1995 and 2005-2010

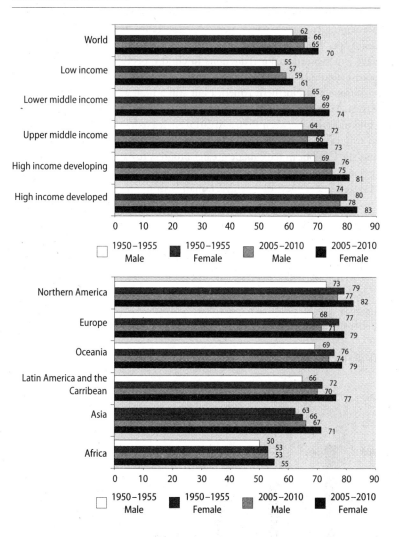

advantage has declined since 1990-1995. In developed countries that trend is associated with reduced sex differences in mortality due to cardiovascular disease and injuries.[6]

⁶ Frank Trovato and Nils B. Heyen, "A varied pattern of change of the sex differential in survival in the G7 countries", *Journal of Biosocial Science*, vol. 38 (2006), pp. 391-401.

A major contributor to the increase in life expectancy has been the decline of mortality in childhood. Globally, mortality under age 5 declined from 233 deaths per 1,000 births in 1950-1955 to 71 deaths per 1,000 in 2005-2010, a 70 per cent reduction. Most of that reduction occurred in developing countries, whose under-five mortality dropped from 271 to 78 deaths per 1,000 between 1950-1955 and 2005-2010. Although all regions have experienced major reductions in child mortality, marked differences persist (figure III). Today, under-five mortality is below 10 deaths per 1,000 in Europe and Northern America but still a high 136 deaths per 1,000 in Africa. Millennium Development Goal 4 calls for a two-thirds reduction in child mortality between 1990 and 2015. Such a reduction is particularly hard to achieve when child mortality is already low. Yet Europe and Latin America and the Caribbean have made greater progress toward that goal than other regions. Declines have been particularly slow in Africa where 4.7 million children under age 5 die each year, mainly from preventable causes.

Because of progress made in reducing mortality at younger ages, the probability of surviving to age 60 at current mortality rates is high, amounting to 79 per cent for females and 73 per cent for males at the global level. As with other indicators of mortality, marked differences exist among major areas and between the sexes (figure IV). At current mortality rates, females have the

Figure III
Under-five mortality by major area, 1950-1955 to 2005-2010

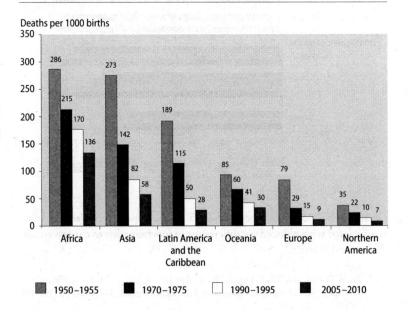

Figure IV
**Probability of surviving to age 60 according to the mortality rates of 2005-2010
by sex and major area** (*percentage*)

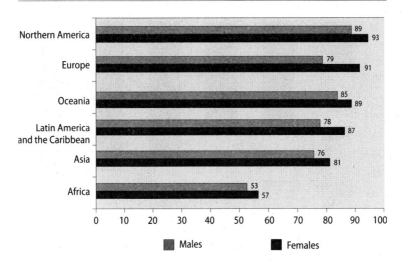

highest probability of survival to age 60 in every region, with particularly high probabilities prevailing in Europe and Northern America (more than 90 per cent). Female chances of surviving to age 60 are also high in Latin America and the Caribbean and Oceania (87 per cent and 89 per cent, respectively). In Asia, they are slightly lower, at 81 per cent, but they are lowest in Africa (57 per cent). Male chances of surviving to age 60 are highest in Northern America and Oceania, at 89 per cent and 85 per cent, respectively; they are lower in Asia, Europe and Latin America and the Caribbean (ranging from 76 per cent to 79 per cent), and particularly low in Africa (53 per cent). That is, even in areas where female mortality is high during the reproductive years, female chances of survival to age 60 are higher than those of males.

As life expectancy rises, deaths become increasingly concentrated at older ages. Thus, at the world level, the proportion of deaths under age 5 declined from 40 per cent in 1950-1955 to 16 per cent in 2005-2010, whereas that of deaths at age 60 or over rose from 26 per cent to 54 per cent between the two periods. Similarly, whereas in Africa today 38 per cent of all deaths occur before age 5, in Europe and Northern America barely 1 per cent do so. Furthermore, in those two major areas, nearly 80 per cent of deaths occur at older ages but in Africa, just 22 per cent of all deaths occur at age 60 or over (figure V).

Figure V
Distribution of deaths by age group and major area, 2005-2010

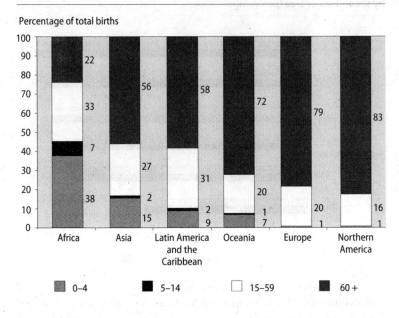

Percentage of total births

Chapter II
Causes of death[7]

The epidemiological transition that underpins the reduction of mortality has produced a major shift in the causes of death. The World Health Organization (WHO) estimates the distribution of deaths by cause according to three major groups of causes. Group I includes infectious and parasitic diseases, respiratory infections, maternal and perinatal conditions, and nutritional deficiencies, that is, it includes all the communicable diseases associated with poverty. Group II encompasses the non-communicable diseases, namely, neoplasms (cancer); cardiovascular, respiratory and digestive diseases; diseases of the genitourinary system; musculoskeletal, skin and oral diseases; diabetes, nutritional and endocrine disorders, neuropsychiatric and sense organ disorders, and congenital abnormalities. Group III includes all injuries, whether intentional or unintentional.

Figure VI
Distribution of deaths by cause and major area, 2004

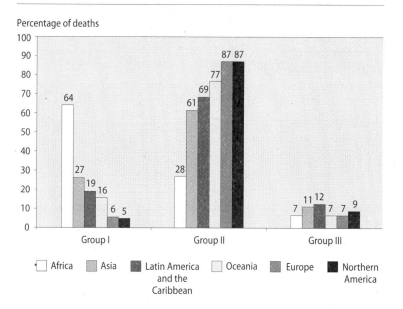

_____
[7] All estimates cited in this section are derived from data presented in *World Health Statistics 2009* (World Health Organization, 2009).

In 2004, 30.6 per cent of all deaths in the world resulted from the causes in Group I, 59.6 per cent from those in Group II and 9.8 per cent from injuries (Group III). The distribution of deaths by cause varied considerably among the major areas (figure VI). In Europe and Northern America, at most 6 per cent of all deaths resulted from communicable diseases (Group I), whereas non-communicable diseases (Group II) accounted for 87 per cent of all deaths. Non-communicable diseases also accounted for the majority of deaths in Asia, Latin America and the Caribbean, and Oceania, with proportions ranging from 61 per cent in Asia to 77 per cent in Oceania. Only in Africa was mortality dominated by communicable diseases: they accounted for 64 per cent of all deaths in the continent.

The causes of death differ by age. In 2004, 89 per cent of the deaths among children under age 5 were caused by communicable diseases as were 53 per cent of those among children aged 5 to 14. Injuries accounted for the other major proportion of deaths among children aged 5 to 14, 30 per cent. Among persons aged 15 to 59, non-communicable diseases accounted for the major share of deaths, 48 per cent, with communicable diseases accounting for a further 29 per cent and injuries for 23 per cent. Non-communicable diseases were the cause of the vast majority of deaths among persons aged 60 or over (86 per cent) and just 10 per cent were due to communicable diseases.

Figure VII
Number of deaths by cause, sex and age group, 2004

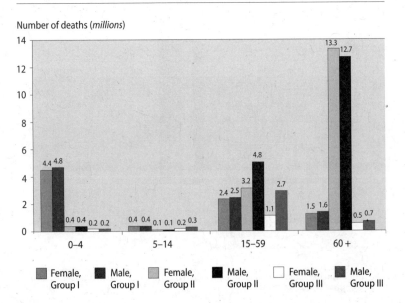

Number of deaths (*millions*)

- Female, Group I
- Male, Group I
- Female, Group II
- Male, Group II
- Female, Group III
- Male, Group III

Figure VIII
Percentage of deaths by cause for major income group, 2004

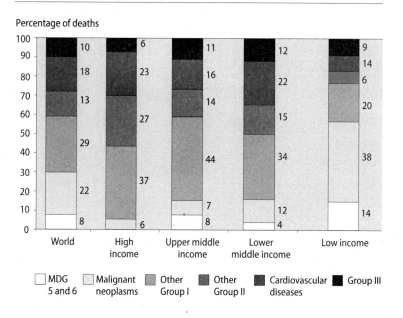

Percentage of deaths

Legend:
☐ MDG 5 and 6 ▨ Malignant neoplasms ▨ Other Group I ▨ Other Group II ▨ Cardiovascular diseases ■ Group III

Data on the number of deaths by cause, age group and sex indicate that at all ages below 60 and for every group of causes, the number of deaths among males surpassed or equalled that among females (figure VII). That finding holds even for the deaths over ages 15 to 59 due to Group I causes, which include those related to maternal conditions. Only among deaths occurring at age 60 or over does the number of female deaths due to non-communicable diseases surpass that of males, mainly because more women than men survive to old age.

The distribution of deaths by cause varies significantly among countries grouped by income (figure VIII). In high- and middle-income countries, cardiovascular diseases account for the largest proportion of deaths, ranging from 34 per cent to 44 per cent. Malignant neoplasms constitute the second major cause of death in high-income countries, but in middle-income countries "other Group II" (non-communicable diseases excluding malignant neoplasms and cardiovascular diseases) account for greater shares of all deaths than neoplasms. In addition, injuries cause double the percentage of deaths in middle-income countries (between 11 per cent and 12 per cent) than in high-income countries (6 per cent). In low-income countries, cardiovascular diseases and malignant neoplasms together account for 26 per cent of all deaths, but their share is markedly lower than the 38 per cent accounted for by "other Group I" (i.e., communicable diseases excluding those covered by Millennium Development Goals 5 and 6). The share of deaths caused by HIV/AIDS, tuberculosis, malaria and maternal conditions (Goals 5 and 6) is highest in low-income countries (14 per cent), followed by upper middle-income countries (8 per cent) and lower middle-income countries (4 per cent). In high-income countries the share of deaths caused by those diseases is virtually nil.

Chapter III
The burden of disease[8]

While the causes of death are indicative of the impact of different diseases on a population, they do not properly reflect a population's health status because many diseases are not fatal and yet reduce the quality of life of those suffering from them. For that reason another measure, the disability adjusted life years (DALYs), is used to reflect both the fatal and non-fatal burden of illness and injury on a population. WHO uses the term "disability" to refer to a "loss of health", where health means having full functional capacity in such domains as mobility, cognition, hearing and vision. The DALYs are the sum of the years of life lost due to premature death and the years of healthy life lost because of disability due to disease or injury.

In 2004, 1.5 billion DALYs were lost by the 6.4 billion people on Earth (see table 1). Low-income countries accounted for 54 per cent of all the DALYs, although their share of the population was just 37 per cent. The lower middle-income countries accounted for 30 per cent of the DALYs, a share lower than that of their population (38 per cent). The upper middle-income countries constituted 9 per cent of the world population and accounted for 8 per cent of the DALYs and the high-income countries, which comprised 15 per cent of the population, produced only 8 per cent of the DALYs. Thus, the global burden of disease was disproportionately heavy on the low-income countries.

At the global level, non-communicable diseases accounted for 48 per cent of the DALYs, communicable diseases, maternal and perinatal conditions and nutritional deficiencies for a further 40 per cent and injuries for 12 per cent. The group of neuropsychiatric disorders accounted for the largest share of the global DALYs (13 per cent) and was followed by cardiovascular diseases and injuries other than road traffic accidents (10 per cent each). Sense organ, musculoskeletal and congenital conditions together accounted for 9 per cent of the global DALYs, the same share as that of HIV/AIDS, tuberculosis, malaria and sexually transmitted diseases combined.

Non-communicable diseases accounted for the majority of the DALYs in high-income countries (85 per cent) and middle-income countries (62 per cent). Both the neuropsychiatric disorders and cardiovascular diseases were responsible for large shares of the DALYs in high- and middle-income countries. Injuries other than road traffic accidents accounted for a major share

---

[8] All estimates cited in this section are derived from data relative to *The Global Burden of Disease: 2004 Update* (World Health Organization, 2008).

Table 1
Distribution of disability adjusted life years according to cause for the world and income groups, 2004

	World	High-income countries	Upper middle-income countries	Lower middle-income countries	Low-income countries
Population (millions)	6 437	977	580	2 465	2 413
Total disability adjusted life years (millions)	1 523	122	121	452	828
			Percentage		
Communicable diseases, maternal and perinatal conditions	39.7	6.0	21.4	22.5	56.6
Non-communicable diseases	48.0	84.8	63.0	61.7	32.9
Injuries	12.3	9.2	15.6	15.8	10.4
Of which:					
Neuropsychiatric disorders	13.1	25.8	16.2	16.6	8.8
Cardiovascular diseases	9.9	14.6	17.7	12.1	6.9
Injuries excluding road traffic accidents	9.6	6.6	12.5	11.9	8.4
Sense organ, musculoskeletal and congenital	9.4	13.2	9.5	12.2	7.3
HIV/AIDS, tuberculosis, malaria and sexually transmitted diseases	9.0	0.8	10.9	3.8	12.8
Neoplasms	5.2	14.9	7.3	7.3	2.4
Road traffic accidents	2.7	2.6	3.1	3.9	2.0
Maternal conditions	2.6	0.5	1.1	1.8	3.5
Diabetes	1.3	3.0	2.1	1.7	0.7
Neglected tropical diseases	1.2	0.0	0.3	0.7	1.9

of the DALYs in upper middle-income countries, which include the Russian Federation, and in low middle-income countries, which include China.

In low-income countries, communicable diseases accounted for the majority of the DALYs (57 per cent) with the share of HIV/AIDS, tuberculosis, malaria and sexually transmitted diseases combined reaching 13 per cent. Nevertheless, non-communicable diseases were responsible for 33 per cent of the burden of disease in those countries and, among them, neuropsychiatric disorders accounted for a high 9 per cent. Injuries other than road traffic accidents accounted for 8 per cent of the DALYs and were followed by sense organ, musculoskeletal and congenital diseases combined and cardiovascular diseases, each with 7 per cent. Maternal conditions accounted for a further 4 per cent of the DALYs in low-income countries, the highest share of maternal conditions among all income groups.

Diabetes accounted for just 1 per cent of the DALYs at the global level but it was responsible for 3 per cent of those of high-income countries and 2 per cent in the middle-income countries. Neglected tropical diseases, which accounted for 1 per cent of the global DALYs, were responsible for 2 per cent of those of low-income countries and 89 per cent of the burden of disease they caused affected people aged 5 to 59, that is, those of school or working age.

At the world level, children under age 5 accounted for 28 per cent of the DALYs in 2004, whereas persons aged 15 to 59 accounted for 49 per cent and persons aged 60 or over for 15 per cent (figure IX). In low-income countries, children under age 5 and persons aged 15 to 59 accounted for 41 per cent and 42 per cent, respectively, of the DALYs. In all other income groups, persons aged 15 to 59 accounted for the highest proportion of the DALYs, followed by persons aged 60 or over. In high- and middle-income countries, children under age 5 accounted for low proportions of the DALYs. Because of the high proportions of older persons in high-income countries,

Figure IX
Distribution of disability adjusted life years by age group for the income groups, 2004

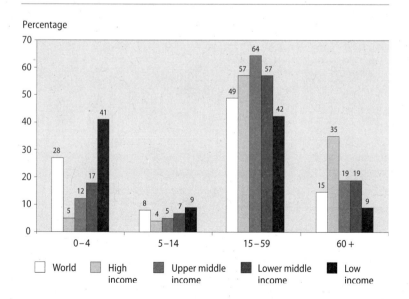

31 per cent of the DALYs in those countries was attributable to persons aged 60 or over. Clearly, major differences in the burden of disease by age are associated with income levels and with differences in the age distribution of their populations.

Chapter IV
Health and development

Better health is associated with higher incomes and better socio-economic status, but the direction of causality remains contested. When estimates of life expectancy for all countries in the world are plotted against GDP per capita, they show an increasing and concave relationship, meaning that, at lower income levels, life expectancy rises faster with increases in income than it does at high levels of income. The shape of this relationship has remained generally stable over time, but the curve has shifted upward on the life expectancy axis, implying that life expectancy has risen without major increases in income (see figure X). By one estimate, just between 10 per cent and 25 per cent of the overall increase in life expectancy between the 1930s and the 1960s can be attributed to increases in income, whereas the rest of the increase was due to other factors, including public health interventions and the diffusion of health innovations.[9]

Figure X
The relationship of life expectancy at birth and GDP per capita, 1980-1985 and 2000-2005

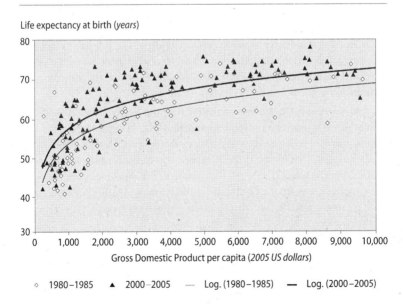

Life expectancy at birth (*years*)

Gross Domestic Product per capita (*2005 US dollars*)

◇ 1980–1985   ▲ 2000–2005   — Log. (1980–1985)   ▬ Log. (2000–2005)

[9] Samuel Preston, "The changing relation between mortality and level of economic development", *Population Studies*, vol. 29, No. 2 (1975), pp. 231-248.

The role of health as human capital and therefore as a determinant of economic growth has increasingly been the focus of attention. It is accepted that, starting in 1800, increases in food supply in today's developed countries produced reductions in morbidity and mortality that increased worker productivity and income growth. Economists posit that longer lives generate incentives to invest in education, increase the time in the labour force and reduce sick time, therefore raising productivity and the income-generating potential of a population. Studies at the individual level[10] have corroborated that health status matters in determining cognitive development, labour force participation, wages and earnings, hours worked, savings decisions and the age at retirement.

Analysis of panel data reveals that education and economic circumstances in childhood are key predictors of health outcomes later in life but the effect on health of an individual's own financial resources in adulthood is less clear cut. It also shows that unanticipated health shocks produce significant reductions in socio-economic status because they reduce a person's capacity to work and lead to income losses.[11] Thus, health both affects and is affected by socio-economic status.

It is not straightforward to generalize the results of studies at the individual level to the national level because of other macro effects related to better health, including positive externalities, such as the effect of health on education, or the diminishing returns triggered by increased population pressure on limited land or physical capital that arise when mortality decreases. Because better health improves cognition and produces incentives to invest in education and education is a driver of economic growth, analyses that incorporate the simultaneous effect of both show that the indirect effect of improvements in health can be significant and positive.

Macroeconomic analysis of the relationship between health and economic growth has taken several approaches. The first uses aggregate economic growth models that incorporate explicitly the effects of health. Such studies suggest that increases in life expectancy can contribute to increasing output, but the effect is stronger if increases in life expectancy are the result of rising life spans among productive workers and weaker if they result from falling infant mortality, which accelerates population growth without necessarily increasing the skill level of the population.[12]

---

[10] M. J. Jusain, "Contribution of health to economic development: a survey and over-view" (2009); available from www.economics-ejournal.org; and M. Suhrcke and others, *The Contribution of Health to the Economy in the European Union* (European Commission, Health and Consumer Protection Directorate-General, 2005).

[11] J. P. Smith, "Unravelling the SES health connection", IFS Working Papers No. W04/02 (Institute for Fiscal Studies, 2004).

[12] M. J. Jusain, op. cit.

The second approach uses regression on cross-sectional data to assess the determinants of increasing income per capita. These studies find a positive, significant and sizeable influence of life expectancy on income.[10] Critics of this approach note that the estimated effects may be biased by the multicollinearity of the variables used and by the effects of omitted variables. To address the problem of multicollinearity, a study[13] used an instrumental variable based on the pre-intervention distribution of deaths by 15 major causes and the dates of global interventions. The study concluded that rising life expectancy accelerates population growth but has only a small effect on GDP, both initially and over a 40-year horizon, largely because land and capital availability does not adjust sufficiently to the accelerated population growth produced by declining mortality. To the extent that the instrument used reflects mainly mortality in childhood, this result is consistent with those produced by aggregate growth models.

An intervention that also affects development, namely, family planning as a component of reproductive health, is not included in the models discussed above. By permitting couples and women to space births and have the number of children they desire, family planning has contributed to reducing maternal mortality and improving child survival. It has also led to reductions in fertility, thus counterbalancing the effect of declining mortality at young ages. Consequently, as economists have shown, it contributes to increasing per capita incomes at both the family and national levels and makes the attainment of both low mortality and low fertility beneficial for development.[14]

The association between increasing socio-economic status and better health is remarkably persistent both among countries and within countries. Even within high-income countries, a health gradient exists whereby people having fewer years of schooling, lower-status jobs and lower incomes have worse health than those placed higher in the socio-economic scale. The more time people live in disadvantaged circumstances, the more likely they are to suffer from poor health. Stress in the workplace increases the risk of disease. These effects are stronger in countries with high levels of inequality. To address the socio-economic gradient in health, a holistic approach that goes beyond health policy is necessary to reduce social stratification, including via labour, education, housing and family welfare policies.[15]

[13] D. Acemoglu and S. Johnson, "Disease and development: the effect of life expectancy on economic growth", *Journal of Political Economy*, vol. 115, No. 6 (December 2007), pp. 925-985.

[14] See E/CN.9/2009/3.

[15] *Closing the Gap in a Generation* (WHO/ER/CSDII/08.1) (World Health Organization, 2008).

Chapter V
The role of primary health care[16]

In 1978, at the Alma Ata Conference, the international community defined primary health care as a strategy that would bring essential health care to individuals and families in the community, as close as possible to where they lived and worked, at an acceptable cost, and that would be an integral part of the health system. The Conference also specified the core components of primary health care as health education; environmental sanitation, especially food and water; maternal and child health programmes, including immunization and family planning; prevention of endemic diseases, appropriate treatment of common diseases and injuries; provision of essential drugs; promotion of sound nutrition; and traditional medicine.

After the Conference, two major approaches to the implementation of primary health care emerged, namely, a selective approach that focused on the most severe public health problems in a community in order to achieve results quickly, and a comprehensive approach that sought to address the overall spectrum of health problems in a community on a long-term basis. The first approach resulted in the development of vertical programmes to address specific health problems through a limited set of interventions. The second approach, described as "horizontal" or "comprehensive", aimed at creating a system of permanent institutions that would foster the active involvement of the community in improving health not just by treating disease but also by focusing on disease prevention and early detection.

Alma Ata's vision has not been easily translated into an effective transformation of health systems and the development of primary health care has stalled in many countries. Over the past 40 years, multilateral, bilateral and private donors have tended to favour vertical programmes for disease control and prevention because they are more likely to produce results over short funding cycles. The expansion of the HIV/AIDS epidemic, in particular, gave added impetus to the vertical approach. Currently, the major international efforts to attain the health-related Millennium Development Goals are based on disease-oriented vertical programmes, some of which have been detrimental to the primary health-care system, with which they compete for scarce human and other resources. Vertical programmes that are not

[16] Based on the *World Health Report 2008* (World Health Organization, 2008); and on J. De Maeseneer and others, "Primary health care as a strategy for achieving equitable care", paper prepared for the Health Systems Knowledge Network of WHO, 2007.

integrated into the general health system also create duplication of administrative costs, lead to gaps in care and undermine the Government's capacity to improve its own health-care services. To avoid these detrimental effects, a code of best practice for disease-control programmes has been developed.[17] The code calls for the integration of most disease-control programmes and activities into health centres offering patient-centred care and into not-for-profit health facilities. It also calls for disease-control programmes to be designed and operated in ways that strengthen health systems and that avoid conflict with health-care delivery.

The development of comprehensive primary health care in developing countries has also been retarded by the underfinancing of the health sector, especially during the period of structural adjustment. In many contexts, the privatization of health services was promoted based on the view, common among donor agencies, that the private sector could deliver services more efficiently than the public sector. As a result, Governments in both developed and developing countries privatized health services, sub-contracted health care to the private sector, leased or sold public hospitals to the private sector or granted managerial autonomy to public hospitals, blurring the boundaries between public and for-profit objectives. These developments, coupled with the increasing specialization of health professionals at all levels (nurses, physicians, public health agents, etc.), have resulted in health systems that provide uncoordinated access to hospitals and fragmented specialist care mainly to those who can afford it. In developed and developing countries alike, public spending in health often benefits the rich disproportionately compared to the poor and people with means consume more care than the poor, who are afflicted by more health problems. Wherever people have to rely on out-of-pocket payments to cover health-care costs, catastrophic health expenses can lead to poverty. In many countries, health services for the poor are highly fragmented and severely underresourced. In addition, the tendency to cluster resources around curative services that tend to be costly leaves insufficient resources for prevention and health promotion activities that, by one estimate, could prevent up to 70 per cent of the burden of disease.

Globally, the share of GDP devoted to health increased from 8 per cent in 2000 to 8.6 per cent in 2005, implying that "the health economy" is growing faster than GDP. Adjusted for inflation, global health expenditure rose by 35 per cent between 2000 and 2005. The rise of non-communicable

---

[17] J. P. Unger and others, "A code of best practice for disease control programmes to avoid damaging health care services in developing countries", *International Journal of Health Planning and Management*, vol. 18 (October/December 2003), pp. S27-S39.

diseases, most of which are chronic and require long-term treatment and management, has contributed to that increase and the high likelihood that the growth of both the burden of chronic disease and health expenditures will accelerate in the future is a major concern in both developed and developing countries.

These developments have prompted policymakers to renew their support for a comprehensive primary health-care approach to counteract the fragmentation of health systems, achieve health equity, promote health security at the community level, and provide a comprehensive and coordinated response to the health-care needs of individuals and their families. To achieve these goals, the primary health-care approach needs to be used as a flexible guiding framework so that it can be adapted to local needs and specific sociocultural contexts. To be comprehensive, primary health care must integrate individual and population-based care by blending the clinical skills of physicians with epidemiology, preventive medicine and health promotion. In principle, primary health care would be part of a district health system and the first point of contact with patients. It would take care of most of the cases presented and direct the rest to secondary- and tertiary-care facilities in a cost-effective manner and while ensuring continuity of care. Interdisciplinary teams, including family physicians, nurses, social workers and nutritionists, would provide continuous, seamless care focusing on health promotion, disease prevention, treatment of acute conditions and the long-term treatment and management of chronic diseases. Through intersectoral cooperation, primary health-care actors would identify community problems affecting health and advocate for solutions.

A comprehensive primary health-care approach can save money. In high-income countries with a strong primary health-care orientation, health expenditure per capita is less on average than in other high-income countries. In addition, maximal access to primary health care with sufficient referral opportunity decreases health inequality.[18] In the United States of America, for instance, higher ratios of family physicians to population are associated with better health outcomes in areas with higher income inequalities. Evidence from developing countries corroborates the potential of primary health care to reduce health disparities. In Mexico, access to primary health-care facilities and continuity of care backed by adequate referral mechanisms have contributed to reducing child mortality in deprived populations.

To institute comprehensive primary health care and reap its potential benefits, a number of reforms are needed. First, there is a need to ensure

---

[18]   B. Starfield, L. Shi and J. Macinko, "Contribution of primary care to health systems and health", *Milbank Quarterly*, vol. 83, No. 3 (2005), pp. 457-502.

that all people have access to primary health care through financing methods that ensure universal coverage and are based on risk-sharing. Second, the delivery of health-care services has to be reformed to ensure that health systems respond to the actual needs of people. Third, Governments must remain committed to undertake public policy reforms so as to integrate public health actions and primary health care. Fourth, leadership in the health field must remain responsive to community needs by encouraging the active participation of community members. The leadership should also work towards improving health through policies in other sectors, including education, food safety and quality, and the control of tobacco and alcohol.

Today, in high-income countries whose health expenditure is high, there is ample room to shift resources from tertiary to primary health care and ensure universal coverage.[19] The challenge is greater but more pressing in middle-income countries, where 3 billion people live and where health systems need to adapt to new demands. In doing so, following a primary health-care approach and ensuring universal coverage are key strategies to avoid the mistakes of the past. Lastly, in the low-income countries, particularly those in sub-Saharan Africa and Southern Asia where 2 billion people live, emphasis on a comprehensive primary health-care approach is essential to ensure health equity. In all countries where universal coverage is not yet a reality, there is a need to shift from reliance on user fees levied on patients to the protection provided by pooling resources and prepayment. Low-income countries, which at present are unable to cover the costs of essential health services, will require external assistance to make the necessary changes.

---

[19] *World Health Report 2008* (World Health Organization, 2008), Introduction and Overview.

Chapter VI
The need for health workers[20]

The health workforce includes all people who provide health services—doctors, nurses, physical therapists, pharmacists, laboratory technicians—as well as management and support workers needed for the functioning of health services. In 2006, WHO estimated that there were 60 million health workers globally, 40 million providing health services and 20 million working in management and other support activities. However, health workers are not equitably distributed neither among countries nor within countries. High-income countries have more health workers per population than other countries. Within all countries, health workers tend to be concentrated in larger cities, while small cities and rural areas face shortages. According to WHO, 57 countries, most of them located in Africa and Asia, lack sufficient health workers to meet the health needs of their populations. In 2006, according to WHO, an additional 2.4 million health service providers and 1.9 million management and support workers were needed by those countries. Those shortages are a major barrier to the achievement of the health-related Millennium Development Goals and make it difficult to develop and sustain the primary health infrastructure needed to reduce inequities in access to health care.

It is urgent to increase investment in the training and support of health workers, including by increasing their salaries and providing incentives to those who work in underserved areas. Assuming that the additional 4.3 million workers needed by the 57 countries facing severe shortages are trained over two decades, health budgets would need to increase by US$ 10 per person per year. In addition to funding, comprehensive plans for the development and maintenance of an effective health workforce need to be drawn up and implemented by committed political leaders. Such plans should ensure that the orientation of health-worker training is appropriate for the contexts in which they will work and that career incentives are included to encourage health workers to serve away from large cities.

In all countries, there is also a need to train existing workers so that they keep up to date with new treatments and practices. Improved management and supervision are necessary to make more efficient use of human resources, particularly in the context of comprehensive primary health care

---

[20] Based on "The global shortage of health workers and its impact", WHO Fact sheet No. 302, April 2006; and "Migration of health workers", WHO Fact sheet No. 301, April 2006.

where new team care models need to be introduced and evidence-based skills for the holistic management of disease need to be imparted. Health workers with advanced communication abilities, able to use techniques to bring about behavioural change and to educate patients, and who have counselling skills are needed the world over to provide care for chronic conditions.[21] Task shifting, whereby highly skilled personnel delegate health-care tasks to less skilled workers who can master them, is also necessary, particularly when, with sufficient supervision and support, volunteers or community health workers can perform those tasks effectively.

Because health workers are in demand in richer countries where salaries are better, health workers from middle- and low-income countries have been migrating to high-income countries. Health systems in some high-income countries have high shares of doctors and nurses trained abroad. Given that people have the right to leave their countries, the cooperation of countries of origin and destination is necessary to reduce the negative impacts of health-worker migration. Countries of origin need to improve the working conditions of health workers, train more and orient training to the circumstances in which they will work (e.g. for rural postings). Donors can provide funding for these purposes. Countries of destination need to train more physicians and nurses locally and should follow responsible recruitment practices. An international code of practice for the recruitment of health personnel has been recently adopted.[22]

---

[21] *Innovative Care for Chronic Conditions: Building Blocks for Action* (World Health Organization, 2002).

[22] *International recruitment of health personnel: draft global code of practice* (A63/A/ Conf. Paper No. 11, 20 May 2010) (World Health Organization, 2010).

Chapter VII

Prevention and treatment of communicable diseases and maternal conditions

Communicable diseases cause 23 per cent of all deaths and 57 per cent of those among children under age 5. Yet most communicable diseases are preventable, treatable or curable with low-cost interventions. It is universally recognized that communicable diseases exact a major toll on the health of the poor and the Millennium Development Goals focus on the prevention and control of the major killers. However, progress towards their achievement is falling short and the Millennium Development Goals do not address all communicable diseases. The key interventions to combat the major communicable diseases, alone or in clusters, are reviewed below.

HIV/AIDS. In 2008, about 33 million people were living with HIV, 22 million of whom lived in sub-Saharan Africa.[23] That year, 2.7 million people became newly infected with HIV and AIDS killed 2 million persons, down from a peak of 2.2 million in 2004. Half of those living with HIV are women and half of new infections occur among young people aged 15 to 24. To prevent the spread of HIV, a multipronged strategy is necessary. It includes education and information campaigns to improve understanding of how HIV spreads and how people can protect themselves, focused programmes to reduce high-risk behaviours, the screening of blood products, preventing the reuse of infected needles, providing access to voluntary counselling and testing to determine who is infected, providing treatment for those who need it and preventing mother-to-child transmission by treating HIV-positive pregnant women. Success in avoiding a generalized epidemic has hinged on reaching high-risk groups, including commercial sex workers, men who have sex with men, and injecting drug users. In countries with generalized epidemics, access to antiretroviral therapy for those who need it has expanded markedly. In 2008, an estimated 42 per cent of the 9.5 million persons requiring therapy[24] were receiving it. Increase in antiretroviral therapy coverage has accelerated thanks to reductions in the price of antiretroviral drugs, such as those negotiated by the Clinton Foun-

---

[23] *2009 AIDS Epidemic Update* (Joint United Nations Programme on HIV/AIDS and World Health Organization, 2009).

[24] HIV infection takes years to weaken the immune system. Therapy is indicated only after there are clear signs of immune system decline.

dation HIV/AIDS Initiative and the International Drug Purchase Facility (UNITAID) in 2007. This effort and the provision of diagnostics will need to be scaled up further and sustained over the long term in order to ensure that people continue to survive with HIV. At the same time, prevention efforts must be strengthened, including by facilitating access to condoms and treating sexually transmitted diseases.

Tuberculosis. In 2007 there were 9.3 million new cases of tuberculosis, 15 per cent of which occurred in HIV-positive persons. If diagnosed early, tuberculosis is curable. Thus, a strategy to eradicate tuberculosis must incorporate both early detection and expeditious use of the Directly Observed Treatment Shortcourse (DOTS) programme, which is highly effective in curing the disease. A growing concern is the increasing prevalence of multidrug-resistant tuberculosis, which affected 3 per cent of newly infected people and 19 per cent of recurring infections in 2007. Both diagnosing this variant of the disease and treating it is costly and demanding. A number of organizations, including the Stop TB Partnership, the Global Fund to Fight AIDS, Tuberculosis and Malaria and UNITAID work to provide drugs for treating drug-resistant tuberculosis.

Malaria. In 2008, there were 243 million malaria cases, which caused 863,000 deaths, four fifths of which were among children under age 5.[25] Nine out of every 10 malaria cases occur in sub-Saharan Africa. Malaria in pregnant women is associated with maternal anaemia and preterm delivery, leading to low birth weight and increased infant mortality. Controlling the spread of malaria involves early diagnosis, effective treatment and prevention of transmission by using long-lasting insecticide-treated bednets and indoor residual insecticide spraying. Because of growing antimalarial drug resistance, in Africa and Asia the only effective treatment for malaria is artemisinin-based combination therapy (ACT), which costs more than drugs that have lost effectiveness.[26] Efforts are under way to scale up ACT treatment, particularly by providing intermittent preventive treatment to pregnant women in high transmission settings and paediatric ACT treatment to children. Expansion of bednet coverage is also being pursued. According to the Roll Back Malaria Partnership, over 700 million bednets need to be deployed by 2010 to dent the spread of the disease.

Neglected tropical diseases. A number of infectious and parasitic diseases, endemic in tropical areas, exact a toll on affected populations by causing chronic morbidity. They include soil-transmitted helminthes (hookworm infection, ascariasis and trichuriasis) and schistosomiasis, all of which

---

[25] *World Malaria Report 2009* (World Health Organization, 2009).
[26] Ibid.

cause anaemia among pregnant women and impair physical and cognitive development in children; lymphatic filariasis, which causes severe leg swelling; trachoma and onchocerciasis, which cause blindness; Chagas disease, which affects the digestive system and heart function; leishmaniasis, which causes skin lesions and ulcers; human African trypanosomiasis (sleeping sickness), and dengue fever, a viral infection. About a billion people suffer from one or more of those diseases or their sequelae.[27] If left untreated, parasite infections can last decades and cause severe disability. They also increase susceptibility to other diseases, including HIV and malaria. Crucially, most of these tropical diseases can be prevented or treated. Access to safe water and basic sanitation reduce the incidence of schistosomiasis and trachoma. Vector control can reduce the transmission of dengue, sleeping sickness and Chagas disease. Single doses of low-cost drugs are effective in treating lymphatic filariasis, soil-transmitted helminthes and onchocerciasis, making possible their control via mass drug administration to affected communities or in schools. Because these diseases are debilitating but do not cause death, efforts to control or treat them are not getting sufficient support.

Communicable causes of child mortality. The main causes of child mortality are acute respiratory infections and diarrhoeal diseases, each accounting for 17 per cent of all child deaths. Vaccines have virtually eliminated pneumonia in developed countries, but are not yet widely used in many developing countries where poverty, inadequate nutrition and indoor air pollution contribute to a high incidence of lower respiratory infections. Improving child nutrition and indoor air quality can reduce the incidence of severe respiratory infections and, when infection strikes, early diagnosis and treatment with antibiotics and oxygen can prevent severe illness and death. A properly functioning primary health-care system would provide such treatment. As for diarrhoeal diseases, their main causes are pathogens transmitted from person to person when faecal matter contaminates water, food or a person's hands. Basic hygiene, including hand washing, and access to safe water and sanitation can dramatically reduce morbidity and mortality from diarrhoeal diseases. When diarrhoea occurs, oral rehydration therapy and zinc supplementation, used in combination with exclusive breastfeeding for infants, nutritional support, and appropriate use of antibiotics, can prevent the progression to severe illness and death. To prevent other major childhood diseases, vaccines have proved successful. Measles, another major cause of child mortality, can be prevented by two doses of a vaccine. In 2007, 82 per cent of children aged 12 to 23 months had received at least one dose of the vaccine. Vaccines are also effective in combating polio, diphtheria,

---

[27] Peter J. Hotez, *Forgotten People, Forgotten Diseases* (Washington, D.C., ASM Press, 2008).

pertussis and tetanus. National vaccine campaigns are examples of vertical programmes that are effective, especially in low-income settings.

Maternal conditions. Although maternal mortality accounts for just about 2 per cent of female deaths worldwide, most of the women who died in 2005 of maternal causes could have been saved if they had had access to appropriate health care. New estimates suggest that maternal mortality has declined from 320 deaths per 100,000 births in 1990 to about 250 deaths per 100,000 in 2008.[28] Virtually all maternal deaths occur in developing countries and about half in sub-Saharan Africa. Despite the progress made in reducing maternal mortality, its level remains unacceptably high in many developing countries. Lack of appropriate obstetric care is the major immediate cause of maternal mortality and morbidity. Globally 300 million women suffer from the sequelae of pregnancy and childbirth and 20 million new cases occur annually. Sequelae include infertility, severe anaemia, uterine prolapse and vaginal fistula. Anaemia, which affects 42 per cent of pregnant women and is often exacerbated by malaria, HIV and other conditions, increases the risk of maternal death from haemorrhage. Globally, 33 million women in developing countries are infertile because of complications from unsafe abortion and maternal sepsis. Assistance from skilled health workers (doctors, nurses or midwives) at delivery is crucial for reducing maternal mortality. In both Southern Asia and sub-Saharan Africa, where the largest number of maternal deaths occur, fewer than half of all births are attended by skilled health workers. To be effective in preventing deaths and addressing complications, skilled personnel must have the proper equipment and be able to refer and transport women presenting complications to emergency obstetric services. Access to such services is still limited in low-income countries. Especially in those settings, providing women with family planning options to avoid mistimed or unwanted pregnancies is a cost-effective intervention to reduce maternal morbidity and mortality. Nearly 53 million unintended pregnancies could be averted annually if the unmet need for family planning in developing countries were satisfied, resulting in the prevention of 150,000 maternal deaths.[29] Provision of both antenatal care and post-natal counselling, education and access to effective contraceptive methods for women who want them are all necessary to improve reproductive health and reduce maternal mortality and morbidity.

---

[28]   Hogan, M.C. et al, "Maternal mortality for 181 countries, 1980-2008: a systematic analysis of progress towards Millennium Development Goal 5", *The Lancet,* published only 12 April 2010, www.thelancet.com.

[29]   Guttmacher Institute and United Nations Population Fund, *Adding It Up. The Costs and Benefits of Investing in Family Planning and Maternal and Newborn Health* (2009).

Chapter VIII
Prevention of non-communicable diseases

As a group, non-communicable diseases already cause 60 per cent of deaths worldwide and 72 per cent of those in middle-income countries, and their share of the burden of disease is expected to increase in the future. Among them, cardiovascular diseases, cancers, chronic respiratory diseases, diabetes and depression represent the leading threats to human health and development. Non-communicable diseases pose a major economic and social burden because most are chronic and require long-term treatment. Yet up to 80 per cent of heart disease, stroke and type 2 diabetes and over a third of cancers could be prevented by eliminating shared risk factors, especially tobacco use, unhealthy diets and physical inactivity. In addition, advances in biomedical and behavioural management have substantially increased the ability of health interventions to prevent and control these diseases, especially when patients receive effective treatments, self-management support and regular follow-up.

As populations age, more people are living with one or more chronic conditions for decades. The increase in sedentary living associated with growing urbanization, the prevalence of unhealthy diets and the global marketing of health risks, such as tobacco, are also factors contributing to that increase. The result is higher demands placed on national health systems and higher health-care expenditures. In addition, because over time adverse risk behaviours tend to become concentrated in the poorer segments of the population, chronic diseases are intertwined with poverty and can, in turn, exacerbate poverty through high treatment costs that need to be sustained over long periods. The increase in chronic conditions in middle- and low-income countries is particularly challenging because many of those countries still have a significant burden of disease from acute infectious diseases, maternal conditions and malnutrition.

National policies in sectors other than health exert a significant and often determining influence in shaping the risk factors for non-communicable disease. Thus, health improvements depend on public policies related to trade, taxation, education, agriculture, urban development, food and pharmaceutical production. Intersectoral action is therefore key in national planning to reduce the burden of non-communicable disease. For instance, changing diets, reducing the prevalence of obesity and increasing physical activity requires achieving behavioural change through changes in food production, marketing and advertising; dissemination of nutritional information; access to health education, and the planning of urban environments and public transportation. In 2004, the World Health Assembly adopted the Global Strategy on Diet, Physical Activity and Health[30] to provide guidance in addressing those factors.

Tobacco use is the single most preventable cause of death in the world since it is a risk factor for all the major non-communicable diseases. While prevalence of smoking has declined in many developed countries and has stabilized or declined slightly among men in much of the developing world, it is increasing among women both in developing countries and in countries of Central and Eastern Europe.[31] Without a sustained decline in prevalence, the number of smokers will increase with the growth in the world population. Because tobacco use is addictive, smokers find it difficult to stop. Therefore, preventing people, especially the young, from taking up smoking is crucial. There is strong commitment among Governments to reduce the spread of tobacco use: as of November 2009, 168 Governments had ratified the WHO Framework Convention on Tobacco Control.[32] The Convention contains provisions for the reduction of both the demand for and the supply of tobacco. Taxing tobacco is one of the most cost-effective health measures that Governments can take.

Small shifts in average levels of risk factors can produce major changes in the burden of non-communicable diseases. Strategies to combat these diseases should aim both at reducing national levels of risk factors and preventing disease in high-risk individuals. Such strategies include changes in laws and regulations; tax and price interventions; advocacy and education; interventions in communities, schools or workplaces; and screening, clinical prevention and disease management. Several elements of these strategies can be implemented even in low-income countries. Intersectoral coordination under a unifying national action plan is necessary to avoid duplication of efforts. The WHO 2008-2013 Action Plan for the Global Strategy for the Prevention and Control of Noncommunicable Diseases provides guidance for action by each of the different actors involved.

To underline the importance of reducing the major risk factors for non-communicable diseases, their specificity in terms of the major components of the burden of disease is discussed below.

Cardiovascular diseases. Cardiovascular diseases account for the largest share of deaths globally: 32 per cent of female deaths and 27 per cent of

---

[30]   Resolution WHA57.17, annex.

[31]   J. Mackay and M. Eriksen, *The Tobacco Atlas* (World Health Organization, 2002).

[32]   Adopted by the World Health Assembly on 21 May 2003.

male deaths in 2004. The biggest killers are heart attacks and strokes, which caused 7 million and 6 million deaths, respectively, in 2004. The major risk factors for cardiovascular diseases are hypertension and high cholesterol levels, which are in turn associated with diets rich in fats and sodium, sedentary lifestyles and tobacco use. The damage caused by diabetes also causes heart disease. High-income countries have reduced rates from cardiovascular disease through a combination of prevention and treatment. Preventive measures include promoting non-smoking environments, healthier diets and increased physical activity, lifestyle changes that have been adopted by important segments of the population. In addition, the systematic treatment of hypertension and high cholesterol has been effective in delaying illness. Nevertheless, the rising levels of obesity and diabetes in much of the world portend increasing difficulties in continuing to reduce the toll of cardiovascular diseases.

   Diabetes. Diabetes occurs when the body does not produce insulin to process glucose (type 1) or cannot use efficiently the insulin that it produces (type 2). Left untreated, diabetes causes high blood glucose levels that, over time, damage the circulatory and nervous systems. In 2004, 220 million people had diabetes and 1.1 million deaths were directly attributable to the disease. Overall, up to 2.9 million deaths may be attributed directly or indirectly to diabetes and its complications, including heart disease and kidney failure. Without proper screening, diabetes very often goes undetected until it has damaged key body systems. Once detected, diabetes and its complications require long-term treatment and continuous management, including through changes in diet and lifestyle. The rising global incidence of diabetes is associated with the increasing prevalence of obesity, particularly in high- and middle-income countries.

   Chronic obstructive pulmonary disease and cancers related to smoking. Chronic obstructive pulmonary disease is a life-threatening lung disease that interferes with normal breathing. In 2004, it caused 3 million deaths, 90 per cent of which occurred in low- and middle-income countries, affecting men and women alike. Because the primary cause of the disease is smoke inhalation, whether from tobacco use or indoor cooking fires, reducing tobacco use and subsidizing the use of cleaner cooking fuels by poor people can prevent the disease. The same is true for the array of cancers most closely related to tobacco use: those of the trachea, bronchus, lung, mouth and oropharynx. In 2004, they accounted for 29 per cent of all cancer deaths and for 34 per cent of those in Asia, excluding Western Asia. Tobacco use is an important cause of excess male mortality. Globally, 80 per cent of smokers are male and the majority of smokers live in developing countries.

   Cancers of the reproductive system. Cancers of the breast, cervix, uterus and ovaries accounted for 18 per cent of all new cases of malignant neoplasms in 2004 and for 13 per cent of the deaths from cancer. Prostate cancer contributed 5 per cent of the new cancer cases and 4 per cent of all cancer deaths. These cancers are the most common among neoplasms in Africa, accounting for 45 per cent of cancer deaths among women and 21 per cent of those among men in that region. Globally, breast cancer is the second most common cancer, accounting for 1.1 million new cases and 520,000 deaths annually, nearly all among women. Early diagnosis of breast cancer improves prognosis and requires mammography screening of women aged 50 to 74. Cervical cancer is the second most common cancer in women worldwide, accounting for about 500,000 new cases and 250,000 deaths annually. More than 4 out of every 5 cervical cancer cases occur in low-income countries and it is the most common type of cancer in Africa and Southern Asia. Mortality from cervical cancer is also higher in the developing world, primarily because effective screening for the disease is rare in developing countries. Cervical cancer is caused by the human papilloma virus (HPV) and a vaccine against it already exists. Some countries have begun vaccination programmes but it is too early to assess their effectiveness. Among men, prostate cancer is the major cancer of the reproductive system and it develops at older ages, with most deaths occurring after age 70. Because it is generally a slow growing cancer, generalized screening is no longer recommended.

Other cancers. In 2004, 64 per cent of cancer cases involved organs other than the lungs or those in the reproductive system. Risk factors for other cancers vary. Overweight and obesity are associated with several types of cancer, including cancer of the oesophagus, colorectum, breast, endometrium and kidney. High intake of preserved meat or red meat is associated with increased risk of colorectal cancer. The composition of the diet is important because fruit and vegetables appear to have a protective effect, decreasing the risk of developing oral, oesophageal, stomach and colorectal cancers. High consumption of alcoholic beverages has been shown to increase the risk of cancers of the oral cavity, pharynx, larynx, oesophagus, liver and breast. Exercise has been found to reduce the risk of colorectal cancer. Certain infective or parasitic agents are linked to cancer: viral hepatitis B and C cause cancer of the liver; the bacterium Helicobacter pylori increases the risk of stomach cancer; schistosomiasis increases the risk of bladder cancer, and liver fluke infection increases the risk of cancer of the bile ducts. Exposure to ionizing radiation can give rise to certain cancers and excessive solar ultraviolet radiation increases the risk of all types of skin cancer. The identification of the different risk factors provides the basis for interventions aiming to reduce their prevalence in the population. Controlling weight and avoiding weight gain in adulthood by reducing caloric intake and by increasing physical activity is protective against cancer. Promoting healthier diets and exercise; vaccinating against hepatitis B; increasing awareness about the dangers of excessive sun exposure, and taxing alcoholic beverages to reduce consumption are all measures that can reduce the incidence of cancer. *Neuropsychiatric disorders.* Globally, neuropsychiatric disorders account for 13 per cent of the disability adjusted life years and depression is responsible for a third of their impact. Despite being important causes of disability, mental disorders do not receive the attention they deserve, particularly in middle- and low-income countries. The stigma that is often attached to mental disorders prevents people from seeking treatment and family doctors are usually not sufficiently trained in recognizing and managing mild to moderate mental disorders. Effective drugs exist today to treat an array of mental disorders and symptom-focused psychotherapies, such as cognitive-behavioural therapy, have proved to be effective in treating certain disorders. To ensure that mental disorders are not disregarded by the health system, health authorities should develop a mental health policy; integrate mental-health treatment into primary health care; budget for workforce development and essential drug procurement, and train primary health-care providers in mental health.

Chapter IX
Preventing injuries

Unintentional and intentional injuries cause more than 5 million deaths each year and several million temporary or permanent disabilities that require hospitalizations, emergency department visits and the use of other health services. While morbidity and mortality from unintentional injuries and violence are public health concerns in all populations of the world, their prevalence and consequences disproportionately affect developing countries where unsafe living and working conditions are common. In 2004, the risk of dying from an unintentional injury was nearly twice as high in low-income and middle-income countries as in high-income countries. Young men are particularly at risk of experiencing unintentional injuries or violence. Eight of the 14 leading causes of death among males aged 15 to 29 in 2004 were injury related, including road traffic accidents, homicides and suicides.

Among the 5.8 million deaths caused by injuries in 2004, road traffic accidents caused 1.3 million. Alcohol use is a major contributor to deaths from both unintentional injuries and violence. The use of alcohol causes 1.8 million deaths annually and 32 per cent of them are from unintentional injuries, many of them involving traffic accidents. In 2004, WHO made recommendations on measures to reduce traffic accidents in the *World Report on Road Traffic Injury Prevention*. Governments are urged to enact comprehensive laws to protect all road users, including pedestrians, by setting appropriate speed limits and blood alcohol concentration limits, and by requiring the use of appropriate protection mechanisms, including helmets, seat belts and child restraints.

Unintentional injuries other than road traffic accidents, such as poisonings, drownings, fires and falls, caused 2.6 million deaths in 2004. To prevent injuries among children, the use of child-resistant containers to prevent poisoning and pool fencing to prevent drowning are recommended. So is the elimination of home hazards to prevent falls, especially among children and the elderly.

Reducing the number of injuries and deaths due to violence requires multisectoral and culturally appropriate strategies. Programmes to restrict access to common methods of suicide and interpersonal violence, such as guns, are effective in reducing mortality from intentional injury. School-based educational programmes to improve self-esteem, control anger and develop appropriate conflict-resolution skills can prevent violence among young people, including between those who are intimate partners. It is also crucial to treat those suffering from depression and other mental disorders and to establish crisis centres that can provide immediate support to victims or potential victims of suicide or violence.

Chapter X
Conclusions and recommendations

The universal decline in mortality that occurred in most countries during the twentieth century has led to life expectancies at or above 69 years in all world regions, except Africa, and to a shift of mortality from the younger to the older ages. Underpinning this transition is the effective control and treatment of the major communicable diseases with the result that, in all world regions, except Africa, they account for moderate to low proportions of all deaths (27 per cent or less). Similarly, their share of the burden of disease is a low 22 per cent in middle-income countries and just 6 per cent in high-income countries.

The decline in the burden of disease attributable to communicable diseases has been accompanied by a rise in that associated with non-communicable diseases, most of which are chronic and require long-term treatment. Among non-communicable diseases, neuropsychiatric disorders and cardiovascular diseases, especially heart attacks and stroke, account for a major share of the burden of disease in high- and middle-income countries. Cancers, chronic respiratory diseases and diabetes are other major contributors to the burden of disease in those countries.

In sub-Saharan Africa, the transition to low mortality had not advanced as rapidly as in other regions by 1980 and the emergence of the HIV/AIDS epidemic slowed down or even reversed in some African countries the gains made during previous decades. Despite the major advances made in reducing the spread of HIV and treating those affected, 2.7 million new cases of the disease still occur annually and, for those receiving treatment, HIV infection has become a chronic condition requiring long-term treatment. Among low-income countries, which include most of those in sub-Saharan Africa and India, 57 per cent of the burden of disease is attributable to communicable disease, including HIV/AIDS, and maternal and perinatal conditions, and an additional 33 per cent is caused by non-communicable diseases. Low-income countries face therefore the double challenge of preventing the spread of communicable diseases and treating those affected while at the same time addressing the growing prevalence of chronic, non-communicable diseases.

In all countries, the poorer segments of the population are more vulnerable to disease and have less means to prevent or treat it. Yet health expenditure tends to favour the rich. Therefore, all countries face the challenge of reducing inequities in access to health care and instituting financing mechanisms that ensure universal coverage based on risk-sharing so as to prevent illness from leading to poverty.

A key strategy in addressing these multiple challenges is to strengthen health systems to ensure that they can deliver the services communities require, including not only curative care and the treatment of acute conditions but also preventive care, health promotion and the long-term management of chronic conditions. A comprehensive primary health-care approach offers a flexible framework to achieve these objectives. To be comprehensive, primary health care must integrate individual and population-based care, blending the clinical approach with epidemiology, preventive medicine and health promotion. It should be the basis of a district health system, with capacity to treat most cases and adequate referral support from secondary- and tertiary-care facilities. It should ensure a holistic approach to health maintenance, disease prevention and the management of chronic conditions through interdisciplinary practice and continuity of care.

A comprehensive primary health-care approach is cost-effective but it can be developed only through a sustained and focused effort over the medium term. For that reason, pressing needs have been mostly addressed through vertical programmes focusing on specific diseases, to the detriment of a comprehensive approach. Because pressing needs are real, health planners and donors need to find novel ways of integrating their interventions into primary health facilities or, when vertical programmes are appropriate, ensuring that they do not adversely affect efforts to strengthen primary health care. In countries depending on donor funding to boost health budgets, continuity of funding is necessary to ensure that efforts to develop a comprehensive primary health-care system are sustained.

A crucial element in the strengthening of health systems is the availability of the necessary health workforce. Shortages of health workers are severe in many low-income countries but they also exist in high-income countries because of the increasing burden of chronic disease among their ageing populations and are growing in middle-income countries. There is a need, therefore, for concerted efforts at both the national and the international level to train an adequate supply of health workers, ensuring that training produces the variety of skills needed and that it is oriented to the contexts in which health workers are required. Devising incentives for health workers to take jobs and remain in underserved areas, especially the rural areas of developing countries, is also necessary. Donor funding can assist Governments of low-income countries to implement national plans on health workforce retention and development. High-income countries should follow responsible recruitment practices in order not to exacerbate the shortages of health workers in low-income countries.

In low-income countries, the current priority is to achieve the health-related Millennium Development Goals and efforts to do so are well under way. Funding for a number of interventions has been growing but is not yet adequate. Scaling up successful interventions is required. The full array of actions needed has been reviewed in the body of this report. One intervention that bears highlighting is support for family planning programmes in the least developed countries. Donor funding for family planning on a per woman basis has declined since the mid-1990s and the unmet need for modern contraception remains high in the least developed countries: one out of every four women aged 15 to 49 who are married or in a union have such an unmet need.[33] By preventing mistimed or unwanted pregnancies, family planning can contribute to reducing maternal mortality by 28 per cent and, by extending inter-birth intervals, it can contribute to reducing child mortality. For every dollar spent in family planning, from 2 to 6 dollars can be saved in interventions to achieve other Millennium Development Goals.[34]

The most cost-effective strategy to reduce the growing burden of chronic, non-communicable disease is to reduce the prevalence of the risk factors associated with the most common diseases. Tobacco use, unhealthy diets, overweight and obesity, physical inactivity and excessive use of alcohol all contribute to raising the risks of the major causes of chronic disease. National policies in sectors other than health exert a significant and often determining influence in shaping those risk factors. Thus, health improvements depend on public policies related to trade, taxation, education, agriculture, urban development, food and pharmaceutical production. Intersectoral action is therefore key in national planning to reduce the burden of non-communicable disease. Guidance on how to improve diets and promote physical activity can be found in the Global Strategy on Diet, Physical Activity and Health adopted by the World Health Assembly in 2004. Provisions to reduce both the demand for and the supply of tobacco are contained in the WHO Framework Convention on Tobacco Control and taxing tobacco is one of the most cost-effective health measures that Governments can take. The WHO 2008-2013 Action Plan for the Global Strategy for the Prevention and Control of Noncommunicable Diseases lists actions appropriate for all actors concerned.

Mental disorders, especially depression, are responsible for an important share of the burden of disease yet mental health treatment is rarely

---

[33] "What would it take to accelerate fertility decline in the least developed countries?" (United Nations Population Division Policy Brief, No. 2009/1).

[34] Scott Moreland and Sandra Talbird, "Achieving the Millennium Development Goals: the contribution of fulfilling the unmet need for family planning" (Washington, D.C., USAID, 2006).

well integrated into the health systems of medium- and low-income countries. Effective drugs exist today to treat an array of mental disorders. To ensure that mental disorders are not disregarded by the health system, health authorities should develop a mental health policy, integrate mental health treatment into primary health care, budget for workforce development and essential drug procurement, and train primary health-care providers in mental health.

Injuries remain a significant cause of death in all groups of countries but exert a heavier toll in middle-income countries. Road traffic accidents account for a fifth of all deaths due to injuries and could be reduced significantly by enacting and enforcing regulations setting appropriate speed limits and blood alcohol concentration limits, and requiring the use of appropriate protection mechanisms, including helmets, seat belts and child restraints. Reducing the use of alcohol and eliminating unsafe housing or working conditions is also important. Restricting access to common methods of suicide and interpersonal violence, such as guns, is effective in reducing mortality from intentional injury.

In sum, if mortality is to continue declining in all countries, the burden of disease will become even more dominated by non-communicable diseases, most of which are chronic and require long-term treatment and management. Since death is inevitable and there are as yet no means of eradicating specific non-communicable diseases, delaying the onset of illness should be the main objective. Fortunately, Governments can do much to achieve that objective, especially by taking measures to reduce the prevalence of risk factors associated with chronic disease. Most of those measures relate to sectors other than health and are cost-effective. Implementing them as soon as possible will buy time to strengthen health systems so as to provide more equitable and effective health care to all those who need it.

ANNEX

Resolution 2010/1
Health, morbidity, mortality and development*

The Commission on Population and Development,

Recalling the Programme of Action of the International Conference on Population and Development[1] and the key actions for its further implementation,[2]

Recalling also the United Nations Millennium Declaration[3] and the 2005 World Summit Outcome,[4] as well as General Assembly resolution 60/265 of 30 June 2006 on the follow-up to the development outcome of the 2005 World Summit, including the Millennium Development Goals and the other internationally agreed development goals,

Recalling further the outcomes of the major United Nations conferences and summits in the economic, social and related fields, especially those related to global health,

Recognizing that the full implementation of the Programme of Action of the International Conference on Population and Development and the key actions for its further implementation, including those related to sexual and reproductive health and reproductive rights, which would also contribute to the implementation of the Beijing Platform for Action,[5] population and development, education and gender equality, is integrally linked to global efforts to eradicate poverty and achieve sustainable development and that population dynamics are all-important for development,

Recalling all General Assembly resolutions related to global public health, including those related to global health and foreign policy,[6]

---

* For the discussion, see chap. II.

[1] *Report of the International Conference on Population and Development, Cairo, 5-13 September 1994* (United Nations publication, Sales No. E.95.XIII.18), chap. I, resolution 1, annex.

[2] General Assembly resolution S-21/2, annex; *Official Records of the General Assembly, Twenty-first Special Session, Supplement No. 3* (A/S-21/5/Rev.1); and A/S-21/PV.9.

[3] See General Assembly resolution 55/2.

[4] See General Assembly resolution 60/1.

[5] *Report of the Fourth World Conference on Women, Beijing, 4-15 September 1995* (United Nations publication, Sales No. E.96.IV.13), chap. I, resolution 1, annex II.

[6] See General Assembly resolutions 63/33 and 64/108.

Welcoming the ministerial declaration of the 2009 high-level segment of the Economic and Social Council, on the theme "Implementing the internationally agreed goals and commitments in regard to global public health",[7]

Welcoming also the Political Declaration and Plan of Action on International Cooperation towards an Integrated and Balanced Strategy to Counter the World Drug Problem, adopted at the high-level segment of the fifty-second session of the Commission on Narcotic Drugs, held in Vienna from 11 to 20 March 2009,[8]

Welcoming further the declaration adopted at the First Global Ministerial Conference on Road Safety: Time for Action, held in Moscow on 19 and 20 November 2009,

Taking note of the decision of the Economic and Social Council to devote the high-level segment of its substantive session of 2010 to the theme "Implementing the internationally agreed goals and commitments in regard to gender equality and the empowerment of women",

Taking note with appreciation of the initiative of the Government of the Russian Federation to organize an international conference on non-communicable diseases in Moscow in June 2011,

Recalling that health is a state of complete physical, mental and social well-being and not merely the absence of disease or infirmity,

Recognizing that population dynamics, development, human rights, and sexual and reproductive health and reproductive rights, which contribute to the implementation of the Programme of Action of the International Conference on Population and Development and the Beijing Platform for Action, empowerment of young people and women, gender equality, rights of women and men to have control over and decide freely and responsibly on matters related to their sexuality and reproduction free of coercion, discrimination and violence, based on mutual consent, equal relationships between women and men, full respect of the integrity of the person and shared responsibility for sexual behaviour and its consequences, are important for achieving the goals of the Programme of Action of the International Conference on Population and Development,

Noting with concern that, despite some progress made in public health in the last decade, for millions of people throughout the world the right of everyone to the enjoyment of the highest attainable standard of physical and mental health, including, inter alia, access to medicines, vaccines and

---

[7]   See *Official Records of the General Assembly, Sixty-fourth Session, Supplement No. 3* (A/64/3/Rev.1).

[8]   See *Official Records of the Economic and Social Council, 2009, Supplement. No. 8* (E/2009/28), chap. I, sect. C; see also A/64/92-E/2009/98, sect. II.A.

commodities, equipment and other supplies and to comprehensive primary health-care services, health promotion and disease prevention, still remains a distant goal and that, in many cases, especially for those living in poverty and populations in vulnerable or marginalized situations, this goal is becoming increasingly remote,

Emphasizing that poverty is a major common denominator in health-related issues and is responsible for the serious worsening, above all in developing countries, of the main health indicators, deterioration of living standards, shortening of the average life expectancy and persistence of, and in some cases, the increase in preventable diseases and deaths, particularly of children,

Expressing deep concern that hundreds of thousands of women die every year from largely preventable complications related to pregnancy or childbirth; that, for every death, an estimated twenty additional women and girls suffer from pregnancy-related and childbirth-related injury, disability, infection and disease; that more than 200 million women worldwide lack access to safe, affordable and effective forms of contraception, and that complications from pregnancy and childbirth are one of the leading causes of death for women between the ages of 15 and 19, in particular in many developing countries,

Noting that, as reported by the World Health Organization, the causes of maternal death, in order of prevalence worldwide, include severe bleeding (haemorrhage), infections, complications due to unsafe abortion, high blood pressure in pregnancy (eclampsia), obstructed labour, and other direct causes, accounting for an estimated 80 per cent of maternal mortality worldwide, as well as other indirect causes,

Emphasizing that achieving the health-related Millennium Development Goals is essential to socio-economic development and poverty eradication, concerned by the relatively slow progress in achieving them, especially in reducing maternal mortality, and mindful that special consideration should be given to the situation in the least developed countries and in Africa,

Noting with concern that perinatal mortality continues to be alarmingly high in many countries, contributing substantially to the lack of progress in the reduction of child mortality and improved maternal health,

Expressing deep concern that some nine million children under five years of age die every year from conditions that are largely preventable and treatable and, in that context, reaffirming the objectives of the Programme of Action of the International Conference on Population and Development concerning the reduction of infant and child mortality, and recognizing the importance of promotion and respect for the rights of the child for the achievement of health-related goals, in particular Millennium Development Goal 4,

Recognizing that communicable diseases, which have been prioritized by the Millennium Development Goals, such as HIV/AIDS, malaria and tuberculosis, as well as other communicable diseases and neglected tropical diseases, pose severe risks for the entire world and serious challenges to the achievement of development goals,

Recognizing also that an epidemiological transition is now under way in all regions of the world, indicating an increase in chronic and degenerative diseases, while high levels of infectious and parasitic diseases persist in many developing countries and countries with economies in transition that are confronting the double burden of fighting emerging and re-emerging communicable diseases, such as HIV/AIDS, tuberculosis and malaria, in parallel with the increasing threat of non-communicable diseases,

Recognizing further that the emergence of non-communicable diseases is imposing a heavy burden on society, one with serious social and economic consequences, and that there is a need to respond to cardiovascular diseases, cancers, diabetes and chronic respiratory diseases, which represent a leading threat to human health and development,

Concerned about the persistence of health inequities, both among and within countries, and gender disparities that have resulted in detrimental health and mortality outcomes and are impeding the improvement of health among women, and noting that such inequities result from economic and social determinants that can be addressed by heeding the recommendations formulated by the Commission on Social Determinants of Health,[9]

Reaffirming that good public health is better achieved through a combination of good public health policies, including multisectoral policies that stress better nutrition, safe drinking water, hygiene, sanitation and sustainable urbanization and that effectively combat major risk factors,

Noting the increase in the prevalence of non-communicable diseases including, inter alia, cardiovascular diseases, chronic respiratory diseases, cancer and diabetes, in all countries and the developmental challenges posed by it, and recognizing the importance of reducing the prevalence of major risk factors for non-communicable diseases including, inter alia, tobacco use, harmful use of alcohol where its consumption is not against the law, abuse of narcotic drugs and psychotropic substances including amphetamine-type

---

[9]   See Commission on Social Determinants of Health, *Closing the Gap in a Generation: Health Equity through Action on the Social Determinants of Health: Final Report of the Commission on Social Determinants of Health* (Geneva, World Health Organization, 2008).

stimulants, unhealthy diets, obesity and lack of physical activity, as identified in the 2008-2013 Action Plan for the Global Strategy for the Prevention and Control of Non-Communicable Diseases of the World Health Organization,

Taking note of the reports of the Secretary-General on health, morbidity, mortality and development[10] and on the monitoring of population programmes, focusing on health, morbidity, mortality and development,[11] and taking note also of the report of the Secretary-General on the flow of financial resources for assisting in the implementation of the Programme of Action of the International Conference on Population and Development,[12]

Reaffirms the Programme of Action of the International Conference on Population and Development[1] and the key actions for its further implementation;[2]

Reaffirms its strong commitment to the full implementation of the Programme of Action adopted at the International Conference on Population and Development in 1994, as well as the key actions for the further implementation of the Programme of Action agreed at the five-year review of the Programme of Action, and the Copenhagen Declaration on Social Development and the Programme of Action;[13]

Recognizes that health and poverty are interlinked and that achieving the health-related goals is central to sustainable development, and encourages Governments to give priority attention to the health-related Millennium Development Goals at the upcoming High-level Plenary Meeting of the sixty-fifth session of the General Assembly;

Encourages Member States and international organizations to scale up actions aimed to accelerate progress on all health-related targets of the Millennium Development Goals, in particular universal access to reproductive health, immunization and key child survival interventions, HIV prevention, mitigation and treatment, prevention and treatment of neglected tropical diseases, prevention and treatment services for malaria and tuberculosis, and access to affordable safe water and sanitation, the achievement of which would have the greatest impact on public health and development;

Reaffirms the values and principles of primary health care, including equity, solidarity, social justice, universal access to services, multisectoral action, transparency, accountability and community participation and

---

[10] E/CN.9/2010/3.

[11] E/CN.9/2010/4.

[12] E/CN.9/2010/5.

[13] *Report of the World Summit for Social Development, Copenhagen, 6-12 March 1995* (United Nations publication, Sales No. E.96.IV.8), chap. I, resolution 1, annexes I and II.

empowerment, as the basis for strengthening health systems, recalls in this regard the Declaration of Alma-Ata,[14] and recognizes the importance of providing comprehensive primary health-care services, including health promotion and universal access to disease prevention, curative care, palliative care and rehabilitation that are integrated and coordinated according to needs, while ensuring effective referral systems;

Recognizes traditional medicine as one of the resources of primary health-care services which could contribute to improved health-care services leading to improved health outcomes, including those targeted in the Millennium Development Goals, and urges States, in accordance with national capacities, priorities, relevant legislation and circumstances, to respect and preserve the knowledge of traditional medicine, treatments and practices, appropriately based on the circumstances in each country, and on evidence of safety, efficacy and quality;

Urges Governments to strengthen health systems so that they can deliver equitable health outcomes on the basis of a comprehensive approach by focusing appropriate attention on, inter alia, health financing, the health workforce, procurement and distribution of medicines and vaccines, infrastructure, information systems, service delivery, planning and implementation, universal access, and political will in leadership and governance;

Calls upon Governments to reduce health inequities by, inter alia, considering the recommendations formulated by the Commission on Social Determinants of Health,[9] and urges the international community to support the efforts of States to address the social determinants of health and to strengthen their public policies aimed at promoting full access to health and social protection for, inter alia, the most vulnerable sectors of society, including, as appropriate, through action plans to promote risk-pooling and pro-poor social protection schemes, and to include support for the efforts of developing countries in building up and improving basic social protection floors;

Emphasizes the need to increase the accessibility, availability, acceptability and affordability of health-care services and facilities to all people in accordance with national commitments to provide access to basic health care for all, as well as the need to increase the healthy lifespan and improve the quality of life of all people, and to reduce disparities in life expectancy between and within countries;

Recognizes, in that regard, the significant efforts undertaken by developing countries, including through South-South cooperation and triangular

---

[14] See *Report of the International Conference on Primary Health Care, Alma-Ata, Kazakhstan, 6-12 September 1978* (Geneva, World Health Organization, 1978).

cooperation, and encourages the international community to enhance support for those efforts;

Emphasizes that advances in health depend, among other factors, on the promotion and protection of all human rights, the promotion of gender equality and the empowerment of women, and the elimination of gender-based discrimination, especially by ensuring equal opportunities for women and men in education, employment and access to social services, including health services; by instituting zero tolerance regarding violence against women and girls, including harmful traditional practices such as female genital mutilation or cutting; by preventing child and forced marriage; and by ensuring women's and men's access to the means to determine the number and spacing of their children;

Urges Governments, in order to ensure the contribution of the Programme of Action of the International Conference on Population and Development to the internationally agreed development goals, including the Millennium Development Goals, to, inter alia, protect and promote the full respect of human rights and fundamental freedoms regardless of age and marital status, including by eliminating all forms of discrimination against girls and women; working more effectively to achieve equality between women and men in all areas of family responsibility and in sexual and reproductive life; empowering women and girls, promoting and protecting women's and girls' right to education at all levels; providing young people with comprehensive education on human sexuality, on sexual and reproductive health, on gender equality and on how to deal positively and responsibly with their sexuality; enacting and enforcing laws to ensure that marriage is entered into only with the free and full consent of the intending spouses; ensuring the right of women to have control over and decide freely and responsibly on matters related to their sexuality, including sexual and reproductive health, free of coercion, discrimination and violence; combating all forms of violence against women, including harmful traditional and customary practices such as female genital mutilation; developing strategies to eliminate gender stereotypes in all spheres of life and achieving gender equality in political life and decision-making, which would contribute to the implementation of the Programme of Action of the International Conference on Population and Development, the Beijing Platform for Action and the Millennium Development Goals;

Urges Governments to redouble efforts to reduce maternal morbidity and mortality by ensuring that universal access to reproductive health, including family planning, is achieved by 2015; that health systems provide a continuum of antenatal and neonatal health care, including delivery assistance by skilled health workers and emergency obstetric care; that women receive nutritional support; and that sexual and reproductive health information and services are integrated into HIV/AIDS plans and strategies;

Also urges Governments to intensify efforts to provide quality delivery care, including during the often neglected early post-natal period, as such care improves health outcomes for both women and children;

Calls upon Governments to scale up significantly efforts to meet the goal of ensuring universal access to HIV prevention, treatment, care and support, and the goal of halting and reversing the spread of HIV/AIDS by 2015, particularly by integrating HIV/AIDS interventions into programmes for primary health care, sexual and reproductive health, and mother and child health, by strengthening efforts to eliminate the mother-to-child transmission of HIV, and by preventing and treating other sexually transmitted diseases;

Notes with concern the feminization of the pandemic of HIV/AIDS, especially among young women, and the fact that women now represent 50 per cent of people living with HIV worldwide and nearly 60 per cent of people living with HIV in Africa and, in that regard, reaffirms the commitment to intensify efforts to ensure a wide range of prevention programmes that take account of local circumstances, ethics and cultural values, such as information, education and communication, as well as encouraging responsible sexual behaviour, including abstinence and fidelity, and expanded access to essential commodities, including female condoms and microbicides, through the adoption of measures to reduce costs and improve availability;

Emphasizes the urgency of combating the main causes of child morbidity and mortality, inter alia, pneumonia, diarrhoea, malaria and malnutrition, through vaccination, long-lasting insecticide-treated bednets, nutritional support, improved sanitation, access to safe drinking water, and access to effective medicines and other treatments, while strengthening health systems;

Stresses the need to sustain and strengthen progress made in combating tuberculosis and malaria and developing innovative strategies for tuberculosis and malaria prevention, detection and treatment, including strategies to treat co-infection of tuberculosis with HIV, multidrug resistant tuberculosis and extensively drug-resistant tuberculosis, including through ensuring the availability of affordable, good-quality and effective medicines and equipment;

Urges Governments to increase efforts to control and eliminate neglected tropical diseases, including through increased use of existing medicines, development of new medicines, research into new modes of vector control, and implementation of appropriate prevention strategies, as well

as to make a concerted effort to eradicate poliomyelitis worldwide by inten-
sifying immunization activities and adopting country-specific strategies to
address the remaining barriers to stopping poliomyelitis transmission, and
emphasizes the importance of strengthening health systems to address communicable diseases;

Also urges Governments to give increased attention to the prevention
and control of non-communicable diseases, further taking into account
the social and environmental determinants of non-communicable diseases
by, inter alia, taking action to implement the World Health Organization
Global Strategy for the Prevention and Control of Non-Communicable
Diseases[15] and its related Action Plan;

Urges Governments to develop and put into effect comprehensive and
integrated illicit drug demand reduction policies, programmes and legal
frameworks, including prevention and care in the health-care and social
services, from primary prevention to early intervention to treatment and to
rehabilitation and social reintegration, and in related support services, aimed
at promoting health and social well-being, aiming to effectively reduce the
direct and indirect adverse consequences of illicit drug abuse for individuals
and all societies as a whole, in compliance with the three international drug
control conventions and in accordance with national legislation;

Emphasizes the role of education and health literacy in improving
health outcomes over a lifetime, and urges Governments to ensure that
health education starts early in life and that special attention is paid to
encouraging health-enhancing behaviour among adolescents and young
people in a gender-sensitive manner, especially by discouraging the use of
tobacco and alcohol, encouraging physical activity and balanced diets, and
providing information on sexual and reproductive health that is consistent
with their evolving needs and capacities so that they can make responsible
and informed decisions in all issues related to their health and well-being
and understand the synergies between the various health-related behaviours;

Underlines the health and rehabilitation needs of victims of terrorism,
encompassing both physical and mental health;

Also underlines its commitment to developing and implementing
national strategies that promote public health in programmes or actions
that respond to challenges faced by all populations affected by conflict,
natural disasters and other humanitarian emergencies, and acknowledges
that inequities in access to health care can increase during times of crisis,
and that special efforts should be made to maintain primary health-care

---

[15] World Health Organization, *Fifty-third World Health Assembly, Geneva, 15-20
May 2000, Resolutions and Decisions, Annexes* (WHA53/2000/REC/1).

functions during these periods, as well as to ensure that the needs of the poorest and most vulnerable are met during the post-crisis, peacebuilding and early recovery stages;

Further underlines the need of people living in situations of armed conflict and foreign occupation for a functioning public-health system, including access to health care and services;

Expresses concern at the continuing increase in road traffic fatalities and injuries worldwide, in particular in developing countries, calls for the implementation of existing General Assembly resolutions aimed at addressing global road safety issues and strengthening international cooperation in this field,[16] and urges Governments to enact comprehensive laws and effective compliance and enforcement measures to protect all road users, including pedestrians, by setting appropriate speed limits and blood alcohol concentration limits, and by encouraging the use of appropriate protection mechanisms, including helmets, seat belts and child restraints;

Recalls the Global Strategy and Plan of Action on Public Health, Innovation and Intellectual Property,[17] and urges States, the relevant international organizations and other relevant stakeholders to support actively its wide implementation;

Reaffirms the right to use to the full the provisions contained in the Agreement on Trade-Related Aspects of Intellectual Property Rights,[18] the Doha Declaration on the Agreement on Trade-Related Aspects of Intellectual Property Rights and Public Health,[19] the decision of the World Trade Organization General Council of 30 August 2003 on the implementation of paragraph 6 of the Doha Declaration[20] and, when formal acceptance procedures are completed, the amendment to article 31 of the Agreement, which provide flexibilities for the protection of public health and, in particular, to promote access to medicines for all, and encourage the provision of assistance to developing countries in this regard; and calls for a broad and timely acceptance of the amendment to article 31 of the Agreement on Trade-

---

[16]   See General Assembly resolutions 57/309, 58/9, 58/289, 60/5, 62/244 and 64/255.

[17]   See World Health Organization, *Sixty-first World Health Assembly, Geneva, 19-24 May 2008, Resolutions and Decisions, Annexes* (WHA61/2008/REC/1), World Health Assembly resolution 61.21.

[18]   See *Legal Instruments Embodying the Results of the Uruguay Round of Multilateral Trade Negotiations, done at Marrakesh on 15 April 1994* (GATT secretariat publication, Sales No. GATT/1994-7).

[19]   See World Trade Organization, document WT/MIN(01)/DEC/2.

[20]   See World Trade Organization, document WT/L/540 and Corr.1.

Related Aspects of Intellectual Property Rights, as proposed by the World Trade Organization General Council in its decision of 6 December 2005;[21]

Encourages all States to apply measures and procedures for enforcing intellectual property rights in such a manner as to avoid creating barriers to the legitimate trade in medicines and to provide for safeguards against the abuse of such measures and procedures;

Calls upon Governments and the international community to develop health workforce strategies and to continue the ongoing work of the World Health Organization on a code of practice on international recruitment of health personnel with a view to its finalization, and to conduct a review of training, recruitment and retention policies in order to provide incentives for health workers to stay in underserved, remote and rural areas, taking into account the challenges facing developing countries in the retention of skilled health personnel, improve the conditions of work and increase the number of health workers to ensure the attainment of the health-related Millennium Development Goals, in particular by training more skilled birth attendants and midwives in low-income countries;

Also calls upon donor Governments and the international community to make international cooperation and assistance, in particular external funding, more predictable and better aligned with national priorities and to channel such assistance to recipient countries in ways that strengthen national health systems; welcomes the progress made in developing new, voluntary and innovative financing approaches and initiatives; and emphasizes that innovative financing mechanisms should supplement and not substitute for traditional sources of finance;

Further calls upon Governments, with the support of regional and international financial institutions and other national and international actors, to adopt appropriate measures to overcome the negative impacts of the economic and financial crises on health, ensuring that policies maintain commitment to the internationally agreed development goals, including the Millennium Development Goals;

Urges Governments to continue to address the environmental causes of ill health and their impact on development by integrating health concerns, including those of the most vulnerable populations, into strategies, policies and programmes for poverty eradication, sustainable development, and climate change adaptation and mitigation;

Recognizes that the lack of adequate funding remains a significant constraint to the full implementation of the Programme of Action of the International Conference on Population and Development, calls upon Gov-

---

[21] World Trade Organization, document WT/L/641.

ernments of both developed and developing countries to make every effort to mobilize the required resources to ensure that the health, development and human rights-related objectives of the Programme of Action are met, and urges Governments and development partners to cooperate closely to ensure that resources, including those from the Global Fund to Fight AIDS, Tuberculosis and Malaria, are used in a manner which ensures maximum effectiveness and in full alignment with the needs and priorities of developing countries;

Reaffirms the need to develop, make use of, improve and strengthen national health information systems and research capacity with, as appropriate, the support of international cooperation, in order to measure the health of national populations on the basis of disaggregated data, including by age and sex, so that, inter alia, health inequities can be detected and the impact of policies on health equity measured;

Requests the Secretary-General to continue, in the framework of the implementation of the Programme of Action of the International Conference on Population and Development, his substantive work on health, morbidity, mortality and development, including integrating a gender perspective into its analyses and recommendations, in collaboration and coordination with relevant United Nations agencies, funds and programmes and other relevant international organizations, and to continue assessing the progress made in achieving the goals and objectives on health, morbidity, mortality and development set out in the outcomes of the major United Nations conferences and summits, giving due consideration to their implications for development.